Lorena Ciullo

HERBA

NO

VERBA

Healer's herbarium

Effective methods of using herbs, for natural healing, health and beauty.

Dedication:

To all the Elsewyns of the world,

who have an erbolaria spirit

and who love Mother Nature,

serving it with a pure and sincere heart.

Healer.

This book was born following the publication of the first novel of the trilogy "Il Monastero delle Erbolarie. The fate of Healer ". You can buy it on Amazon:

You can follow me on Facebook

Lorena Ciullo scrittrice

You can follow me on Instagram

Lotain66

You can follow me on the site

lorenaciulloscrittrice.com

Dear Elisewyn,

I'm in my new cell at the Academy and I miss you so much already. I don't know anyone, except the monk Daryus, who accompanied me here, and I don't even know how long he'll stop.

The Academy is in all respects the same as the Monastery, but situated under the waves of the Northern Ocean. We have come this far, entering a cave, guarded by Malachias - a winged and faceless creature - and walking along a very steep tunnel. The entire Academy is protected by a gigantic transparent crystal dome and we breathe thanks to the machines, which inject air from the outside and make an infernal noise. I don't understand how you could wish to live in this unnatural place. I already feel nostalgia for the warmth of the sun and the air perfumed by flowers.

Here, too, they have managed to make herb gardens and plantations, but their scent and their colors seem faded and non-existent. I continue to live this adventure, without knowing where it will lead me, and not having you close, it makes my soul full of fear and melancholy. After the daily lesson, there are three places where I take refuge and find a little comfort. The kitchens, where I eat with the attendants, who are very kind to me; the laboratory, where I compile records for the monk and my cell, where I study. It is from my cell, which I am now writing to you. The classroom where the lessons are held is entirely attended by boys, herbalist apprentices and future monks. As you already know, I am the only girl admitted to the courses and have been relegated to the left wing of the classroom. The boys, on the other hand, are all in the right wing, crammed into the benches and don't even give me a glance. They are totally invisible to their eyes. It is not that this disturbs me, on the contrary. I prefer their indifference, to blame and to the little treats that the Magister Beithin reserves for me, when from time to time he looks at me.

This evening, while I was studying, you came back to me, sweet Elisewyn, with your disarming smile. I thought about how much you wanted to be here now, in my place and learn everything that I find myself forced to study. So I decided to write this Erbolario for you, which I hope will one day deliver to you, making you a welcome thing. Parchments are one of the few things that abound in the Academy. Writing this manuscript will be a consolation for me and a way to honor your sweet memory, dear friend. A way to feel closer, in this time lived alone and in trepidation. Hoping to see you again soon, I remember you with all my affection and my respect.

your Healer.

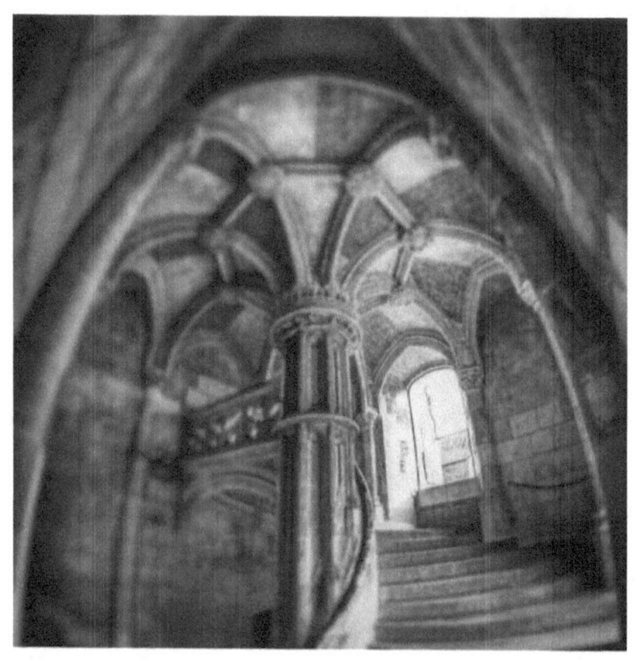

The Academy, where Healer is forced to study, and where he writes the Manuscript.

AROMATIC AND MEDICINAL HERBS

In this section of the manuscript I will write to you about herbs and their characteristics. You already have a lot of knowledge about it, but I think it will be useful to know more.

Nature is full of resources and we manage to catch only a small part of it, the one we need to heal ourselves and get better. We should actually expand our knowledge on the beneficial effects of plants, not only for our well-being, but also to honor a Mother, so generous for her gifts.

Here in the Academy, everything is done to get more intensive than necessary every year, because the Monastery can make more profit.

There is a waste and an exploitation of plants and soil, which sometimes I believe they no longer have the right energy to interact with our bodies and heal them.

As you already know, plants are living beings and they also suffer silently from mistreatment and impoverish themselves for exploitation. If only we understood that it is all a question of fragile balance, this life of ours on Earth, blessed by the love of Mother Nature!

Believe me Elisewyn, sometimes I think the Academy is a great torture room for these poor plants, forced to be born and grow in a crystal vial, under the ocean and us with them.

In this manuscript I will bring back to you the information I am studying at the Academy and I will compare it with what, instead, we erbolarie know from our millennial tradition. Knowledge, passed from hand to hand and from mouth to mouth, thanks to the care and dedication of the Mothers. I entrust them to you, so that your maternal instinct can be fertilized by an immortal seed, the seed of love and the custody of that great gift, which is Nature.

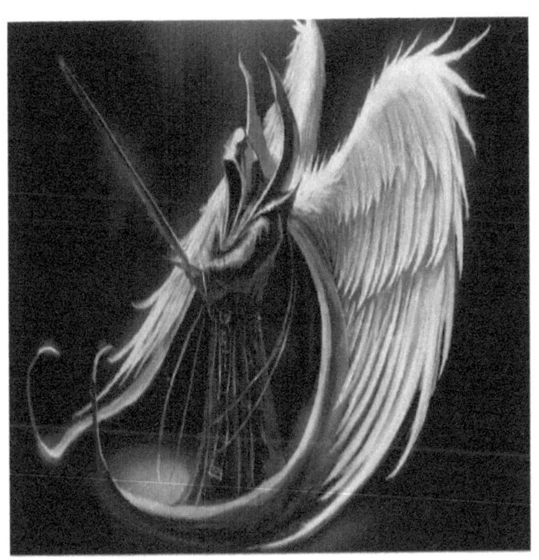

Malachias, was the celestial creature placed by Asmodeus, the Dark Abbot, to protect the cave, which was the entrance to the Academy.

Garlic

The origins of garlic are lost in the mists of time.

It is a bulbous, which is cultivated with ease. Ground between November and December, the bulb tolerates both frost and drought well. Even if the elves call it "fetid rose", in reality neither do they despise its properties.

Here in the Academy garlic is considered more for its exorcistic properties than for its therapeutic properties. In fact they teach that garlic can drive away spells, witches and even demons. Here the cultivation is all destined to the production of crowns to be resold in the villages. There is a large trade in the disclosure of fear and the Dark Abbot has made it one of his biggest income. The women of the villages hang these wreaths at the entrance door, to keep away the evil and its evil spells.

In reality garlic has many properties, so much so that for us erbolaria is considered as a remedy for a hundred illnesses.

Garlic shredded on children's dishes, purifies their intestines, which bring their hands into the body every day, bringing germs into the body to no end. Besides being an excellent wormer, garlic counteracts jaundice and cures asthma. Furthermore, the use of this little friend of nature effectively promotes diuresis, counteracts poison and purifies the skin of juvenile sebum. It is the best vaccine against infections and gives men great sexual vigor.

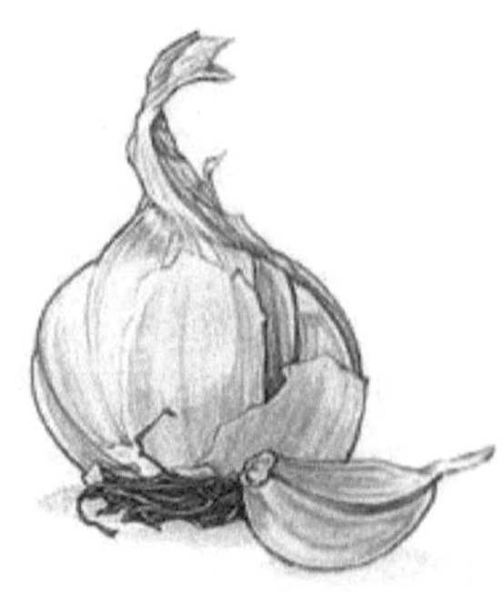

In his small chest the most powerful antidote to tumor formation is hidden. It counteracts cholesterol, because it burns fat in the fluid, which nourishes our body. In this way it prevents heart attack and stroke.

As you will understand, garlic is our ally and should be consumed in the right way.

In fact, being an excellent fluidifier, it also helps lower pressure.

If you don't consume it just because it leaves an unpleasant smell in your breath, know that that aroma doesn't come from the underworld, as they teach here in the Academy, but from a mineral called sulfur that has beneficial effects for the respiratory tract and the bronchi.

A remedy exists for us to remedy halitosis caused by garlic. After eating a clove of garlic, we chew some coriander seeds.

Even if the garlic doesn't taste good, it's worth eating one clove a day, for all the benefits I've listed so far. Do not you think?

LAUREL

Laurus Nobilis, not to be confused with *Lauro Ceraso*, is a plant rich in properties.

Laurel is an evergreen shrub, with shiny and oval leaves, to which the greatest health benefits are attributed. It is a rustic species that adapts to any type of climate and can be grown in any type of garden or vegetable garden. It grows spontaneously, especially in the woods and in the hilly areas.

The properties of the laurel are due to its rich content of essential oils, present in the berries and leaves. As you already know, laurel leaves can be harvested throughout the year, but they are particularly rich in beneficial principles and aromatic essences, from winter to spring.

The berries are harvested between October and November, when they take that beautiful dark color.

The herbalists of the Academy cultivate laurus nobilis, exclusively to make crowns to be placed on statues of deities, invented by the Dark Abbot and for ritual use. In fact they believe that, by burning dried laurel leaves, they can drive away evil spirits and give honor to the deities, present in the Abbey of the Monastery and in the chapels of the villages.

We Herbolaria honor this sacred plant, which offers us beneficial substances for the treatment of many diseases. Substances such as eugenol and limonene are present in the leaves. We consider them beneficial for their antiseptic, antioxidant, digestive and anticancer properties. Fresh laurel leaves are a very important source of vitamin C. In fact 100 grams of fresh laurel leaves contain 46.5 milligrams of ascorbic acid, about 77% of recommended daily doses. As you know, ascorbic acid is one of the best natural antioxidants, able to counteract free radicals. The same acid also stimulates the immune system and healing.

Nelle foglie fresche è presente anche l'acido folico. In 100 grammi ne contengono 180 milligrammi. L'acido folico è importante per la sintesi del Dna e nel corso della gravidanza previene la comparsa di difetti del bambino alla nascita. Le foglie contengono anche la vitamina A, che protegge dal cancro ai polmoni. Sono presenti anche le vitamine del gruppo B, che regolano il metabolismo, contribuiscono alla sintesi di enzimi e al funzionamento del sistema nervoso.

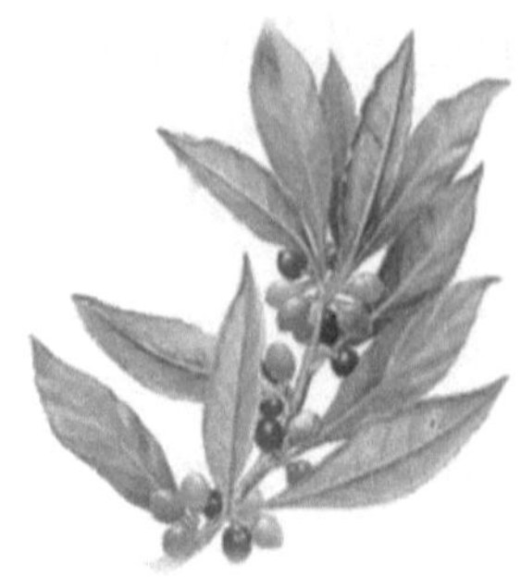

In bay leaves, a true deposit of minerals such as potassium, copper, calcium, manganese, iron, selenium, zinc and magnesium. Potassium is important for keeping blood pressure and heart rate under control. Iron is necessary for the production of red blood cells. The components present in the bay leaves are used for the production of medicines for the treatment of arthritis, muscle pain, bronchitis and flu symptoms.

Calendula

Calendula Officinalis, dear Elisewyn, is a precious plant for its innumerable properties. Its name originates from different meanings. It would seem to indicate the first day of the month, and therefore indicates that it blooms at the beginning of each month throughout the summer period. Another meaning that is observed here with the title of "Solis Sponsa", ie Bride of the Sun, means that this flower opens its corolla at sunrise and closes it at sunset. Surely it will have to do with the stars, since the seeds that are made from it, are in the shape of a lunar quarter. However, it is a wonderful flower that brightens my heart.

At the Academy they have classified about twenty species of this plant, but the one used for medicinal therapies is called Calendula Officinalis.

As I wrote to you, Calendula Officinalis has many healing properties with antispasmodic and healing effects. For example, the decoction of Calendula Officinalis is effective for gastric ulcers and mucosal ulcers. It has sweating effects when you have a fever and prevents menstrual pain, regularizing the flow. The erbolaria use calendula, mixed with other herbs, to combat the annoying alteration of the mucous membranes of the nose.

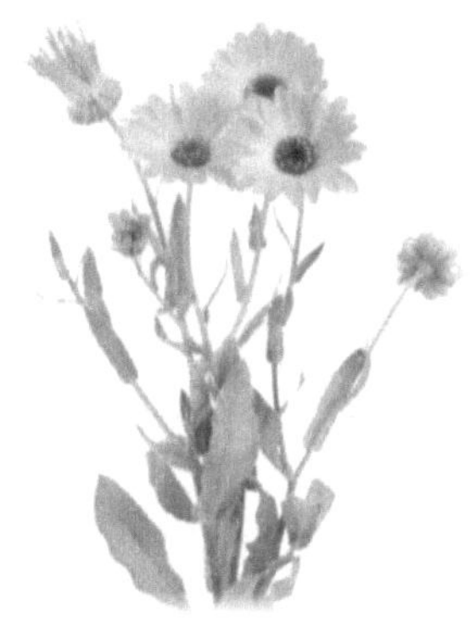

Of great benefit are the ointments and oleolite, which is made to treat burns, dental care and postpartum. Calendula oil is an oil obtained from the maceration of flowers in a carrier oil. It has a powerful eudermic action, because it is able to improve the condition of the skin. Its use is useful whenever the skin is chapped or irritated.

Calendula oil is also a great ally of mothers. In fact it soothes and protects the sensitive and delicate skin of babies and children. Furthermore, if used in a preventive way, it counteracts the formation of fissures at the breast of the nursing mother, and is able to heal those already present quickly.

With the calendol oleolite it is also possible to make the calendula cream excellent for erythema, eczema and sunburn. Likewise, soothing calendula butter is an excellent skin repairer.

Calendula mother tincture is a product that should never be lacking in homes.

It has a soothing and anti-inflammatory action for acne, mild dermatitis and mycoses.

For "external uses" we erbolarie recommend it as:

Refreshing and softening action. It is an excellent cure for chilblains and sunburn, but also effective for candidiasis and vaginitis.

Scarring action for abrasions and insect bites or jellyfish. Excellent for decongesting the mucous membranes of the mouth and calming gingivitis.

15-30 drops diluted in a glass of water will be sufficient to make local compresses with sterile gauze or rinses of the oral cavity.

For "internal use", the mother dye performs:

An antispasmodic action, for pains

abs,

calms and regulates menstrual flow;

a calming and decongestant action for the throat;

an emollient action for the mucous membranes, ideal in the case of colitis, gastric ulcers or internal inflammations;

a digestive action, for those suffering from slow digestion;

hypotensive action, for those with high blood pressure.

For "internal use" 10 to 40 drops are recommended for 2 or 3 times a day, depending on the case to be treated, prolonging the therapy for about two months.

I remind you that marigold flowers are edible, therefore edible, when they are

fresh. You will be able to decorate dishes and thus color a good bowl of rice or a nice cake.

Cypress.

The cypress exercises beneficial activities towards the microcirculation, in this case of hemorrhoids and peripheral venous insufficiency. Last but not least the cypress carries out an anti-inflammatory action for the respiratory system.

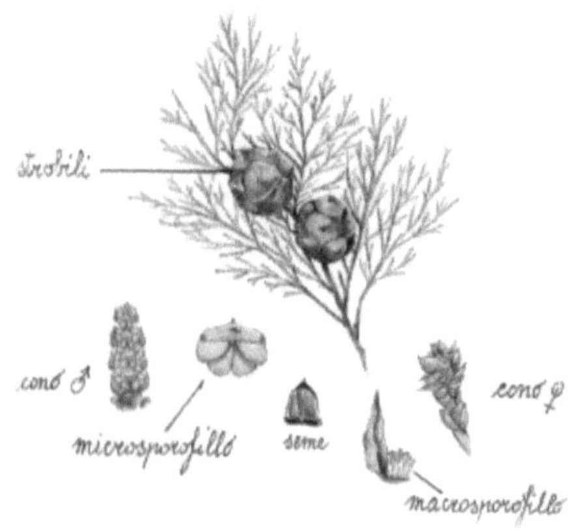

The use of the cypress itself is not allowed here in the Academy, although we then find it mixed for other preparations and needs. Thanks to substances called polyphenols it has astringent, constrictive and antispasmodic properties. It also has beneficial effects on cramps and a sense of swelling in the legs.

The cypress essential oil has anti-inflammatory properties in the respiratory tract, as well as balsamic, expectorant and sedative properties for cough. Thanks to the presence of diterpenes, cypress oleolite is effective in slowing joint osteoarthritis. The use of this plant must however be contained because an abuse could lead to renal irritation.

Turmeric

Turmeric is also called the "spice of miracles". This is thanks to curcumin, the active ingredient of a plant rich in properties. The part that is rich in benefits is the root. Curcumin is a polyphenol with powerful medicinal properties. Turmeric improves the immune defenses and in particular the antiallergic ones. It is also a natural pain reliever. It is able to pass joint and inflammatory pains.

It acts against cell aging. Furthermore turmeric protects the liver, gastric mucosa and intestines.

It stimulates appetite, cures ulcerative colitis and fights eye inflammation.

Turmeric acts as a support for blood production, regulates blood circulation and is an excellent adjunct to the cardiac, circulatory and nervous systems. For these reasons it also has an impact on preventing neurovegetative diseases such as Alzheimer's, Parkinson's and multiple sclerosis.

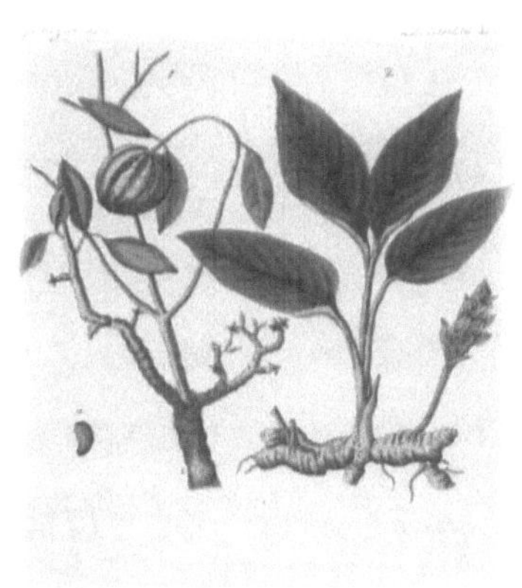

Horsetail

A plant that ignores existence in the Academy is horsetail. Instead, it is known among the erbolaria for its healing and regenerative capacity of nails, hair and joints. It is also an excellent ally to promote diuresis.

The active ingredients of horsetail are: silica, calcium, magnesium and potassium. Thanks to these minerals, horsetail contributes to the "bone metabolism" and promotes remineralization of the osteo-articular system and hard tissues, such as nails and hair.

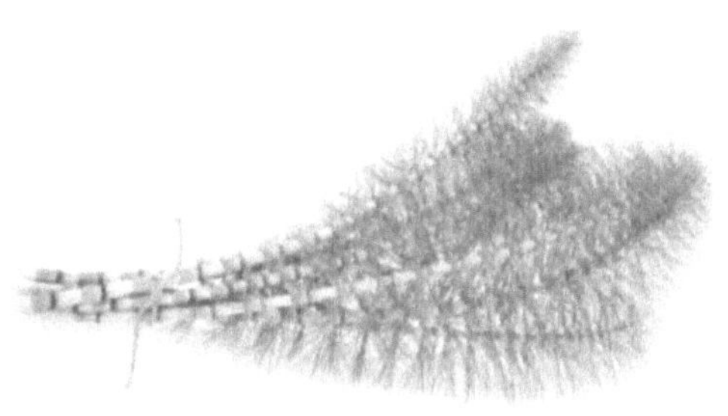

Its intake is therefore indicated in case of nail fragility, hair loss, alopecia, osteoporosis, arthrosis, sequelae of fractures and tendinitis.

The horsetail or ponytail is also an excellent diuretic, therefore indicated for a treatment of metabolic waste.

It is a capilloprotector due to its astringent property on blood vessels, useful against capillary fragility.

HEATHER

The heather or Calluna vulgaris is also known by the name of Brugo, from here moorland. It is a small perennial shrub. Calluna comes from the Greek Kallyno which means to clean. In fact, the name refers to the use of branches, which were used to make sweeping brooms.

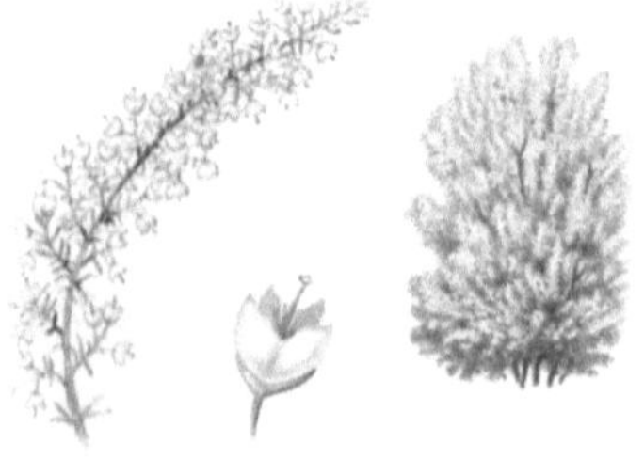

It is an officinal plant with a diuretic, antirheumatic, antiseptic, anti-inflammatory action. Contrasts cystitis because it eliminates urea, uric acid and organism toxins.

Heather is used against water retention or for patients suffering from obesity, who have a greater need to eliminate toxic substances.

Heather also has slightly sedative properties, due to the presence of flavonoids, useful against insomnia.

Different parts of the plant are used. The flowers have an astringent and antiseptic action, while the branches of the plant have anticancer properties.

With heather it is possible to make decoctions, and mother, oleolite and glycerine macerate dyeing. The decoctions are valid as toning for the muscles and should be used in the bathtub.

The proportions are 2 grams of grass for a cup of water. Leave to simmer for about 10 minutes.

The mother tincture is used as an antibacterial and diuretic. Just 30 drops in a little water. The heather oil is useful against skin inflammation; while macerated is used for cystitis and urethritis. In this case it takes just 50 drops in a little water to be taken three times a day. Avoid using the heather in case of liver failure. Too high doses can irritate the intestine.

fennel

Wild fennel, called fennel, is an aromatic plant and is part of the Umbelliferae family, whose name "Foeniculum Vulgare Miller".

The seeds are rich in interesting active ingredients for the functionality of the stomach and intestines.

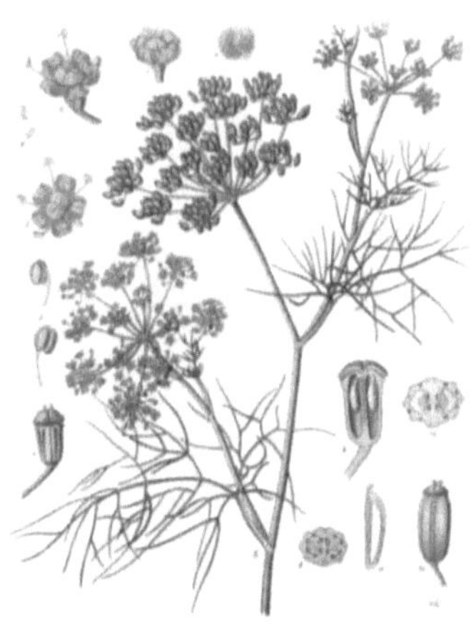

Wild fennel has carminative properties: it absorbs and eliminates intestinal gases, caused by poorly digested foods. It has antispasmodic properties and eliminates gastrointestinal colic and digestive difficulties. It also has diuretic properties, therefore helps to deflate the body from excess fluids and facilitates diuresis.

The herbal tea made with wild fennel together with dandelion, milk thistle and artichoke, sublimates the detoxifying and diuretic effect. The use of wild fennel eliminates catarrh and bronchial affections, freeing the upper respiratory tract. Furthermore, the warm infusion of wild fennel in the evening, before going to bed, promotes a peaceful rest.

"The aromatic and medicinal herbs have properties, which must be discovered in the daily attendance of nature". Healer.

Lavender

Lavender is one of the most popular plants in the garden as well as being one of the oldest. The inflorescences are rich in linalool, responsible for the main therapeutic properties of the plant. It has a sedative, rebalancing action, of the central and vegetative nervous system, digestive, antiseptic and anti-inflammatory.

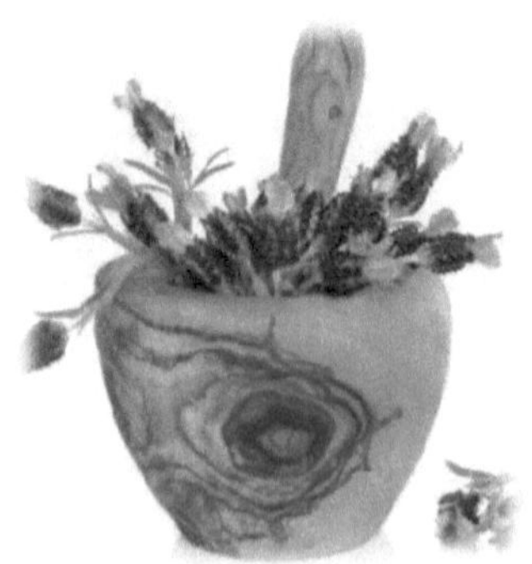

Lavender calms rheumatic pains of joint and muscle origin,

applying the essence, oleolite or lavender water.

Wounds washed with a lavender herbal tea helps to quickly heal wounds and ulcers. Finally, the oil helps relieve the pain of insect bites and spiders.

The essence has balsamic properties: taken for inhalations it accelerates the treatment of laryngitis, pharyngitis, bronchitis and bronchial catarrh and colds.

The scent of lavender reduces anxiety and emotional stress, reduces headaches. Aromatherapy with lavender improves sleep quality.

Lavender essential oil cleanses the skin, brightens it and reduces pimples and acne. A drop behind the ears or behind the neck is an excellent prevention against pediculosis. In addition to being pesticide, it neutralizes the venom of the viper bite. It is a rejuvenating skin and restores the right balance to cutaneous sebum in the hair.

Finally a few drops of lavender in the diffuser perfume the rooms of the house, improving the family harmony. If children find it difficult to sleep, a nice bath with a few drops of lavender oil or a massage with lavender oil would be effective.

Mandrake

Dear Elisewynn, here we enter the darkest mystery of the use of plants. As you know officially in the Monastery as well as in the Academy, it is strictly forbidden to use the Mandragora, because it is considered a magical and demonic plant.

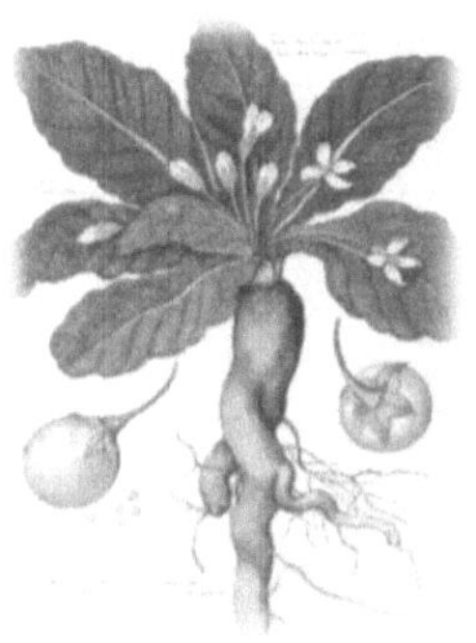

Actually we erbolarie, we use from the beginning. I won't deny that you have to handle it with great care as it is not without side effects.

The Mandragora officinalis or Atropa mandragora is part of the solanaceae family and the shape of its roots resembles that of the human body.

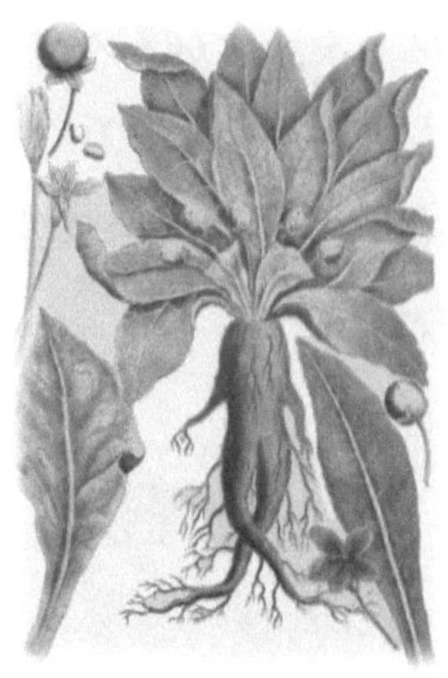

It is probable for this anthropomorphic aspect, that in antiquity the plant was the object of great fear and trembling.

Among the main properties of Mandragora is the ability to induce a state similar to that of the REM phase of sleep. For some active ingredients the plant has narcotic and sedative power. It also has a strong aphrodisiac potential.

Since it is a highly toxic plant, we erbolarie take precise information from the Mother, whenever we have to use it for the cesarean or other operations.

Rosehip

In an erbolaria garden you cannot miss the dog rose. Known in all the Lands for its orange-colored berries, which are a particularly rich source of vitamin C and bioflavonoids.

Excellent combination for the absorption of this vitamin with all its benefits.

The first characteristic of the dog rose is the ability to be immunomodulatory, ie it is able to balance the functioning of the immune system and regulate it according to the needs of the moment.

Excellent as a preventive treatment or in the early stages of flu, cold and cough.

Another property is its being anti-inflammatory. For this reason it is used for allergies and rhinitis. Used to counter cough and cold, it brings great relief to the patient. Because the berries are rich in ascorbic acid, they have astringent and therefore excellent properties in case of diarrhea.

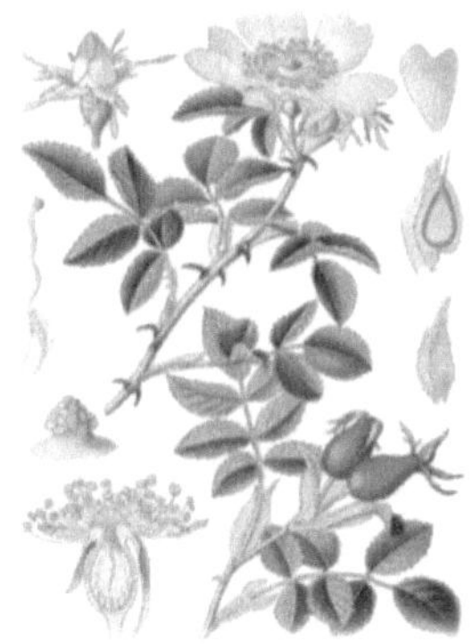

Finally it tones the body of those who take daily portions of rosehip berries.

Excellent intake during periods of psychophysical stress and fatigue. It is a sweet diuretic, because it does not stress the kidneys, while it helps them expel toxins from the body through urine.

The dog rose can be taken both fresh and dried, taking into account, however, that the high presence of vitamin C is present in fresh berries.

The use of wild rose during pregnancy and lactation is not recommended.

Rosemary

Rosemary is a plant rich in essential oils, flavonoids, phenolic acids and tannins, resins, camphor and even rosmarinic acid, which has antioxidant properties. It can be used as an infusion and decoction. Excellent for the proper functioning of liver activities. For this reason it is used together with dandelion and burdock in herbal teas.

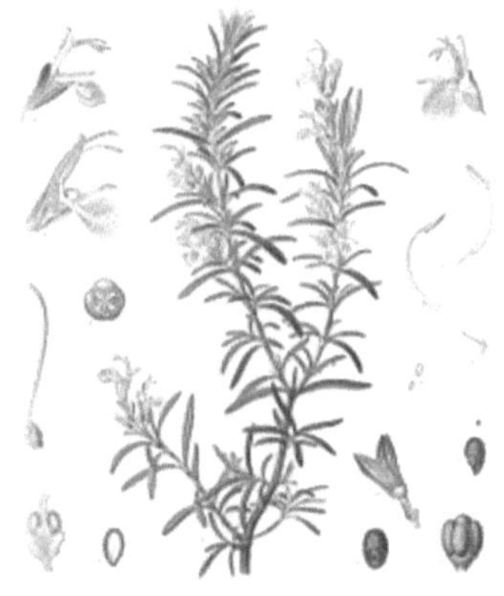

It has balsamic properties and is therefore excellent for coughs, fever and colds.

According to our studies rosemary stimulates an energizing action of the body and mind. Mixed with mint and sage it offers an aphrodisiac effect.

For external use, it is excellent for gingivitis, rheumatism and headache. Valid to rinse the hair, because it stimulates the peliferous follicles, preventing hair loss and favoring regrowth.

The use of mother tincture facilitates psychophysical reinvigoration. Thirty drops in a little water, two or three times a day, give benefits to the bronchial tubes, promote

digestion, help the circulatory
and diuretic system to function
properly.

Sage

Sage leaves include bitter principles, phenolic acids, flavonoids and an essential oil containing thujone, cineol, linalool, beta-caryophyllene and many other substances.

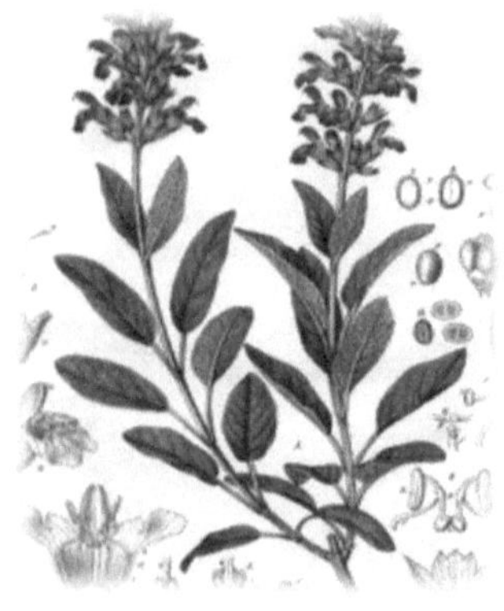

Flavonoids perform an estrogenic action. Sage is used for all female disorders, such as premenstrual syndrome and menopausal disorders.

Since the essential oil stimulates the female hormonal system, it promotes menstrual flow and regulates it. In the essential oil there are also antiseptic properties, which fight catarrhal forms and inflammation of the throat, cold and fever.

Sage is also used in gastrointestinal diseases, as it acts as an antispasmodic. Carnosic acid and triterpenes give sage anti-inflammatory and diuretic properties, offering a good response against water retention, edema, rheumatism and headache. Sage prevents blood sugar spikes.

An infusion of this herb, on an empty stomach, is effective for lowering the glycemic level.

Sage has beneficial effects for the stomach, promotes digestion and fights gastroesophageal reflux.

So sage is an excellent ally for women and for those suffering from excessive sweating and inflammation of the tonsils. It seems to have a good influence on memory, cognitive activities and mood.

lime

In my land, in the Kentrix, there is a grove of fragrant lime trees. Their birth is lost in the mists of time. Very long-lived trees, ideal for making those who insist never fall in love open their hearts to feelings of love and self-giving.

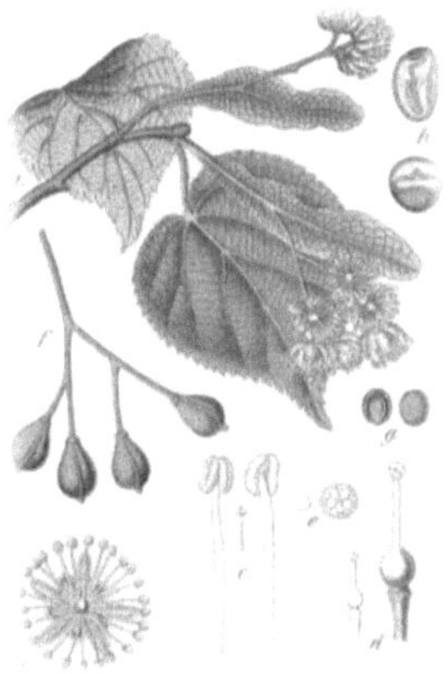

The linden with its leaves and its flowers offer the erbolari the solution for insomnia, thanks to the presence of tannin, flavonoids, essential oils and mucilage. These substances also cure anxiety and tachycardia, headaches and stress, because it plays a relaxing action on the circulatory system, causing a lowering of pressure.

Linden is the most suitable plant also for disorders of the airways of children and adults, because the mucilage contained in the flowers, confer mucolytic and anti-inflammatory properties, effective in case of cough and phlegm.

Excellent antispasmodic for gastrointestinal disorders and irritable bowel.

Linden is also a symbol of conjugal love. It is told how a married couple, who died in mysterious circumstances, her husband turned into an oak, while his wife into a splendid specimen of lime. Elisewynn remembers, the linden is a sacred tree, and as such it leads the erbolari towards truth and harmony.

thyme

The name Timo comes from an ancient language, which means courage, strength. In fact, the twigs were burned and the warriors were incensed before going into battle.

It is a powerful remedy for coughs, whooping cough and respiratory distress. Often the thyme here in the Academy is used for culinary purposes, however this plant has great therapeutic powers.

Especially when the coldest months of the year are approaching, and the cold is pressing, whoever has thyme with him can feel comfortable. Thyme essential oil, called thymol, inhibits the development of bacteria and viruses.

The essential oil of thyme extracted with steam distillation is distinguished by its intense and spicy aroma.

Erbolaria use thyme from the dawn of time for many ailments, such as inflammation of the throat, rheumatic pain, headache, laryngitis, gastritis and digestive disorders.

For external use it is applied on wounds with compresses to disinfect the damaged part. It has no contraindications as an aromatic herb, but if you have intolerance it can cause nausea and vomiting.

Verbena

Verbena is a spontaneous plant rich in beneficial properties. It is suitable for multiple applications. The properties the plant is known for are: anxiolytic, anti-stress and calming. It is recommended in case of severe stress and panic attacks. Its sedative property is also functional for cramps, insistent coughing and muscle strains.

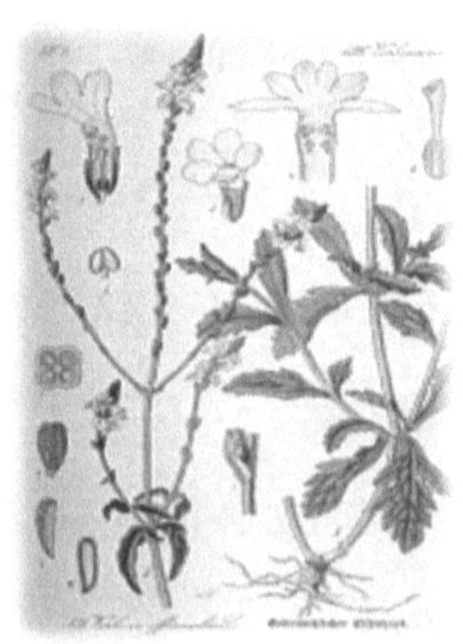

Thanks to the verbena we can cure: sinusitis, asthma, abscesses, arthritis, burns and itching. The effective properties for urinary tract problems should not be forgotten; liver and kidney problems; eliminates intestinal parasites and rebalances thyroid functions.

Verbena essential oil has the ability to rebalance mood and relieve stress layers there are several ways to alleviate it, anxiety, apathy, fatigue, nervousness and insomnia.

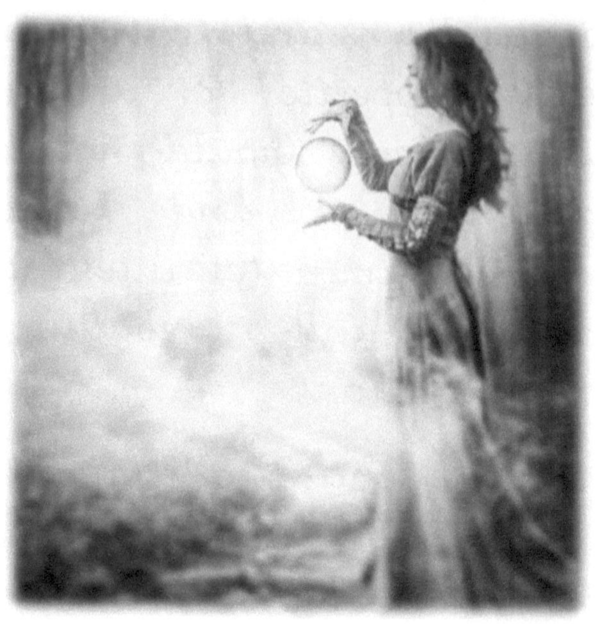

"Knowing and getting into the balance of nature shows you the way to wellness and health".

Healer

EXTRACTIONS

Introduction

Dearest Elisewynn, the time has come that perhaps you are waiting with great trepidation, the moment to learn effectively the use of herbs in the various ways of transformation. Infusions, herbal teas and decoctions are not all the same thing. Each has its own peculiarity and a specific procedure. Sometimes there is a lot of confusion about how to prepare and take the active ingredients that are good for us. Here's how not to make mistakes.

Infusions

Usually the tea is to use the leaves and flowering tops of a single grass, chosen for its properties.

Preparation.

It is poured directly the boiling water over the herbs and covers the cup or pot with lid, for an infusion time that varies depending on the active principle that we want to extract, from 10/15 minutes to an hour. It must then be drained without compressing. The amount will be a teaspoon of tea drugs for a cup of boiling water.

The infusion can have a more or less bland action. It can be concentrated or diluted and drunk throughout the day.

The herbal teas

Although the tea is a fairly new method is the way to take the active ingredients of the most popular herbs. The herbal tea provides a mixture of herbs: one that represents the basic remedy, the second aid that the properties of the first remedy in a synergistic way and the third to serve as a flavoring agent, to improve the taste.

Preparation

Before taking herbs undergo a husking, then they are finely chopped and sieved to remove dust. The mixture must be homogeneous for the preparation time, no more than 10/15 minutes. As nell'infuso pouring the boiling water over the herbs and the pan is covered with a lid. Then it down without squeezing.

The proportions will be 10/20 grams of mixture per liter of water. Even the tea can be drunk throughout the day.

The decoction

The decoction is the beverage which is obtained by extracting the active ingredients through the boiling of the hard parts of plants, such as roots and seeds. Unlike the previous two cases, the herbs are boiled with water.

Preparation.

They must crush the herbs with a pestle before you boil them, so that you will release the active ingredients. The boiling time depends on several herbs used.

It is important to follow the recipe for non-oxidizing substances or even remove harmful ingredients of the plant.

oleolito

The oleolito or macerated oil is the result of a process where you soak the plant in a vegetable oil, said carrier oil. In this way, the fat-soluble components of the plant will be released in the oil, enriching useful for massage substances, ointments, creams.

So the first thing to do is to see if the plant is fat-soluble, or water-soluble if it is possible to make a tincture.

To make a oleolito you need to choose a carrier oil heat resistant and therefore with a very low risk of rancidity.

The best oils are rice oil and grapeseed because poorly marked resistant and smell.

Even olive oil is a heat-resistant oil, but has a sharp odor and could cover one of the herbs.

Sunflower oil and sweet almond are cheaper, but they are much less heat resistant. Vice versa is great jojoba oil, and the only flaw is the very high price. My oleolites I make them with rice oil.

Preparation.

First you need the drug to be added to the oil carrier.

It is appropriate to choose it dry, to prevent rancidity of the oil for the presence of fresh water in the grass. The only exception is for the St. John's wort oleolito, one has to do with the fresh plant.

The oleolito you can do with one or more drugs. For capacities there are no fixed rules. The important thing that put grass in the jar, to be fully submerged oil. Instead there is to say about the various types of oleolito.

We have the cold digestion. In an airtight jar is placed the coated drug with oil and let soak in the dark for 30-40 days, moving the content once every two days, to avoid the formation of mold.

There is also the hot digestion. In an airtight jar it places the covered drugs of oil and let soak in the sun, covered with aluminum foil. For instead hypericum sunlight must hit directly the jar. The exposure time is 15 days.

With fresh herbs it is also necessary to eliminate the deposits of water released from the plant, so as not to ruin the oil.

Finally we digestion in a water bath. In an open jar lies drugs covered in oil and left in a water bath with a very low heat for about three hours.

Finally we have the filtering. I may want to filter in two stages. In the first through a sieve to filter the bulk of the drug, squeezing and thus obtaining the greatest amount dell'oleolito; the second part you do with gauze or a cotton handkerchief, to eliminate even the smallest impurities.

Even the conservation of the oil is very careful. Once ready the oleolito you have to store in an airtight jar away from direct light and heat sources.

The one you can keep for about two years.

Tincture

Make a tincture can be done, but it is always advisable to contact the erbolaria Mother for a product complies with the standards. However, I'll explain how you can do.

The plants should be washed accurately and with clear water. Ensure that the proportions are correct. The proportion is 50 grams of herbs for 10 cl of alcohol.

Cut the plants into small pieces, put them in a sealed container and fill it with alcohol up to completely cover the plants.

Mix the solution and let it sit for three weeks in a dry, dark place.

After the exposure time can strain the liquid and recover the mother tincture. Write the date of production. This dye will be valid for five years. With dried herbs active ingredients will be less strong.

THE RECIPES

Sage infusion

The infusion of sage can be prepared both with fresh leaves that with those dried. With the latter dose it is less because it is stronger. How to proceed? When you are using fresh sage, you will need to put 8/10 well washed leaves of sage and private stem, per cup. If the leaves are dry, just a teaspoon, ie the quantity of a tea bag.

Put water in the pot and make heat on the stove. As soon as the water has reached the boiling temperature, pour it over your leaflets, which are in a cup.

Now wait 3/5 minutes for the Macerino leaves perfectly.

If you want a more intense flavor you can keep to infuse for

7-8 minutes. If you want you can add honey and lemon.

Laurel infusion

To achieve a good bay infused take of green leaves and leave them whole. Proceed as for the infusion of sage. Boil the water, and place the leaves in the cup.

Pour the water on the leaves and leave to infuse for 5-7 minutes. You can sweeten with honey.

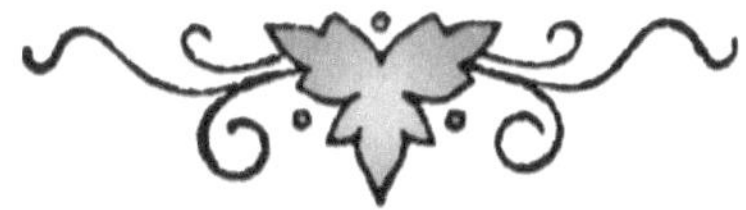

Rosemary infusion

Put water on to boil. Prepare a tablespoon rosemary leaves. Just stamp salt water, pour it in the bowl and leave to infuse for 10 minutes. You can sweeten with honey.

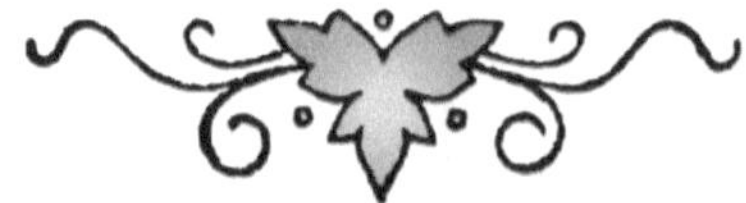

Post sbronza infusion:

If you treat a headache after a hangover of mead or other strong drink, that's the right infusion for you.

Put two teaspoons of St. John's wort in the cup and pour the water after reaching a boil. Leave on for at least 10 minutes. Filter and drink the brew.

Thyme cough inhalation

In cases of coughs, thyme inhalations can help thanks to its anticonvulsant effect and expectorant.

Just put one or two tablespoons of thyme in two liters of boiling water. He puts a towel on the head and inspire the steam with long, deep breaths, until you feel the need.

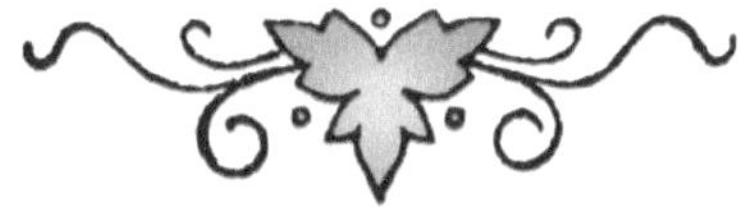

Thyme infusion

Against the spasmodic cough, cold or flu. Versa a teaspoon of thyme in a cup with 250 ml of boiling water. Leave to infuse for 5 minutes and filter it into another cup.

To soften the cough, add a teaspoon of honey. To drink without sugar if you suffer from an upset stomach.

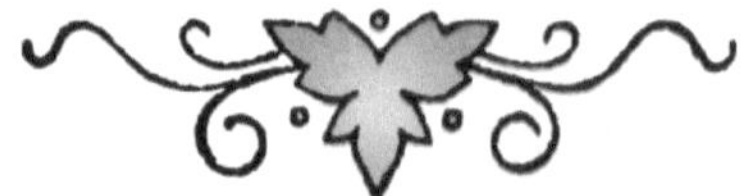

Herbal tea to strengthen hair

Following the infusion procedure, put in the same proportions: rosemary, thyme, lime, sage and marjoram. Drink this tea every day. With the same preparation every night can rub the scalp with a cotton pad. This way you'll have scoured and strengthened hair.

Herbal tea vs influences No. 1:

To counter the cold, and speed up your metabolism, thus obtaining a slimming effect. Put infusion ginger, cinnamon and a bit of a teaspoon honey.

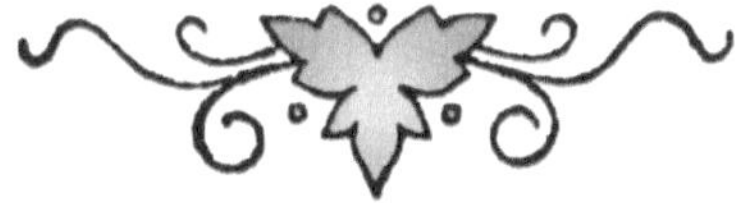

Relaxing herbal tea:

To promote a restful relaxing, take a teaspoon of chamomile flowers, half a teaspoon of lavender flowers food, that has not developed as camphor, and a rosebud dried. Pour the boiling water into the cup and allow to steep for 15 minutes.

Herbal tea digestive:

A teaspoon of chamomile flowers, three teaspoons of cloves, half a cinnamon stick or a tip of a teaspoon of cinnamon powder. Leave to infuse at least 15 minutes.

Herbal tea vs flu n° 2:

To combat seasonal ills. Two slices of fresh ginger, a teaspoon of dried mint, a teaspoon of mauve flowers. Leave to infuse 15 minutes.

Herbal tea a load of energy:

A pinch of cinnamon stick and half, half a teaspoon of green tea, three cardamom pods, 1 or 2 black peppercorns. Leave to infuse for 15 minutes.

Herbal tea for dark circles and puffy eyes:

Remember to drink. Dark circles and puffy eyes are a problem elimination of toxins. Alterna water in unsweetened tea, a blend of dandelion, artichoke and fennel. The three herbs taken in three equal parts, mixed and put into the cup.

When the water boils, pour and leave on for 15 minutes. Filter and drink when it's warm.

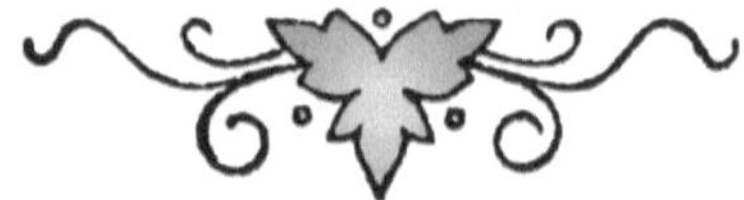

Decoction against back pain:

To prepare the tea with turmeric put to boil a pint of water. Reached the boil plunges a turmeric root peeled and cut into pieces. Let boil for 10 minutes. Lights off the heat and leave to infuse another 10 minutes. Filter the contents and drink two cups a day.

Decoction for endocrine system:

Parsley balances the endocrine system and is effective for those suffering from hypothyroidism.

In a saucepan, add 150 ml of water and 6 grams of dried parsley root. Turn and brings to a boil.

Simmer for 10 minutes. Then Lights off and leave on for another 10 minutes. Filter and edulcora with honey. Excellent as a diuretic, reducing water retention and swelling of the abdomen and legs.

Calendula oil:

Take a sterilized glass jar. Enter dried marigold flowers to three-quarters of the jar and cover with carrier oil to the beginning of the can neck.

The oil in fact, must cover the flowers, but must not touch the cap. Merge twenty drops of essence of lavender, which will help the transmigration of the essential oils of calendula carrier oil. Close the cap and place the jar in a dry, dark place.

Move the contents every two days. Leave on for 30/40 days. I may want to put a note of the dates of beginning and end of the transformation process. The past 30 days, open the jar and filters. A first time passes the oil into a sterilized container with the colander.

The second time you do with the aid of a sterile gauze, to remove any form of impurities.

With this oil can make even the cream butter and calendula.

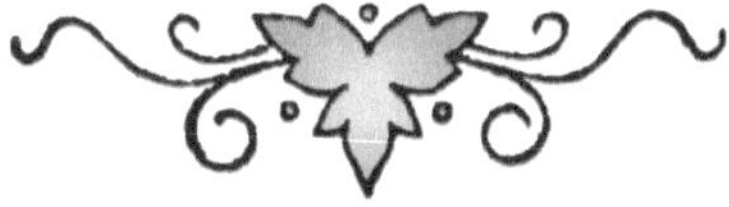

Calendula cream.

To make an ointment Calendula is necessary:

56 grams of distilled water

20 gr of helichrysum hydrolat

3.5 grams of Glycerin stearate

0.3 grams of xanthan gum

15 drops of lavender essential oil

10 drops of rose essential oil.

Preparation:

Stir in a pyrex glass vessel distilled water, the hydrolat helichrysum and xanthan gum. In another glass container together with the oleolito calendula and the emulsifier the glyceril stearate. Place the two containers in a water bath until the emulsifier is melted. Pour the oil phase (oleolito and glycerin) in the aqueous phase (hydrolat helichrysum and xanthan gum).

Stir vigorously to obtain an emulsion. When the mixture will be creamy and thick add the essential oils and the preservative (five drops of vitamin E, tocopherol), not to go rancid cream. Keep at room temperature for three months in a dry and dark place.

Marigold butter:

50 grams of calendula oleolite

25 gr of shea butter

25 grams of mango butter

Preparation:

Melt in a double boiler shea butter and mango butter. When the mixture is liquid remove it from the water bath and add the oleolito marigold.

Amalgam the ingredients well. Transfer the mixture into clean and sterile jars and let cool at room temperature for a few hours. Keep the butter in a cool, dark place. Burn it within two three months.

Cypress oil:

250 grams of pampering

500 ml of carrier oil

1.5 ml of non-acetate tocopherol vitamin E, because that acetate is not antioxidant.

Preparation:

The cypress oil is prepared using the berries, better known as cuddles. These must be collected when they reach their maximum size, around February - March, and they must still be green. In these conditions they will break more easily and release a very good resin scent.

Wash the cuddles, the cypress berries, and after having dried them with a pestle cloth enough to open them and then allow the oil to penetrate. They don't have to get mush. Put them in a previously prepared pot for bain-marie cooking. Prepare with the hot procedure to avoid mold due to the presence of water in the cuddles.

Cover the berries with oil without putting the lid on. Fill the larger pot with water and insert the small one with the berries in it.

Simmer the water for three to four hours. The boil must be sweet and the water level must be equal to or higher than that of the oil. Add water to maintain the same level. Sometimes the berries turn to help the water evaporate.

Finally turn off and let the oil cool. Filter the oil with a sterile gauze and a funnel. Do not wring gauze at the end,

to prevent the pulp from falling into the oil. Observe if any parts of the water have remained in the oil. Keep the bottle turned over overnight.

If there is water it will thicken in the neck of the bottle. You will have to remove it gently (I unscrew the cap and leave it attached to the mouthpiece. The first thing that will come out will be the water. To avoid the risk of losing the oil, put a container ready to recover even the oil). Finally add 10 drops of vitamin E or ROE rosemary oleoresin. Bottles and preserves in a cool and dry place.

CONCLUSION

Dear Elisewyn,

this is the information that I was able to gather in my living room in the Academy. I hope you can come in handy. I will enter this brochure in the bag of monaco, that I may take it when you have to return to the monastery. I enclose with herbarium a big hug, hoping to see you soon. Much more I want to teach you the knowledge of erbolarie, which is already within you, as in every living being. You just need someone to help you see the kaleidoscopic beauty of nature within you and come into harmony with it. Make good use of the herbs and always for a beneficial purpose.

Pray, praises and thanks, but with that song you from the

heart and not as an empty
ritual, just as it does in the
Monastery of Herbalists.

your Healer.

Author's note.

This manuscript was present at the time of the fire in the Monastery of Herbalists. Elisewyn, he found in his cell slightly burnt.

Applications for Elisewynn to Healer: "Why is not burned completely? Because only the edges? "Healer so he explained the strange phenomenon.

The purifying fire has burned every thing belonging to the Abbot Dark and his guild. Reached the manuscript has also started burning, feeling that the scrolls came from the Academy.

But when it came to the name of erbolarie and, primarily that of Healer, has set back its tongues *of fire, preserving the manuscript.*

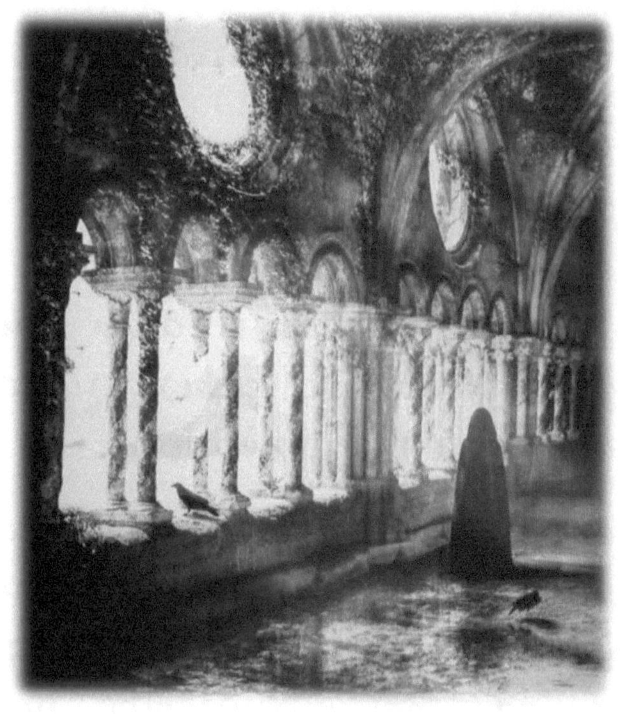

Healer, in the Monastery of Herbalists.

Now it's up to you. What recipes have you found?

Here you can write your info on other aromatic and medicinal plants. Draw the parts of the plant that you have discovered useful for your psychophysical and spiritual well-being.

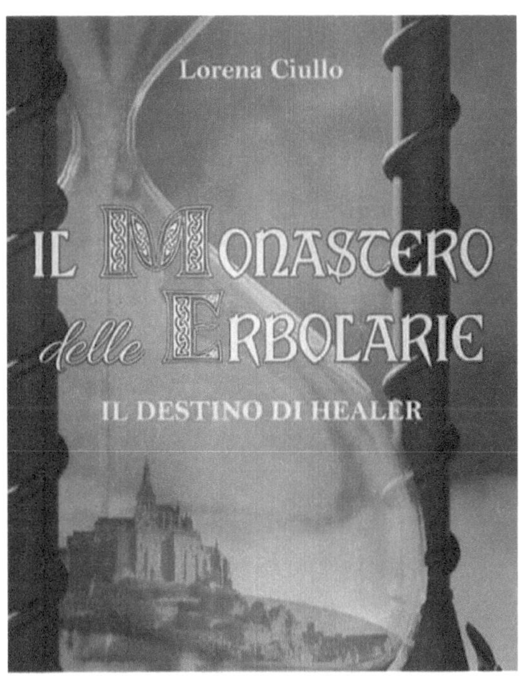

The novel, where the manuscript originated and soon can also buy it on Amazon in English.

www.ingramcontent.com/pod-product-compliance
Lightning Source LLC
Chambersburg PA
CBHW031300250726
48655CB00005B/2287